Day 22,732

A Cancer Survivor's

Guide to Living

Kenneth Edward Ballard

Dedication

To my wife Rissa, the only love of my life. Thank you for walking this walk with me. Please wait for me. You know where.

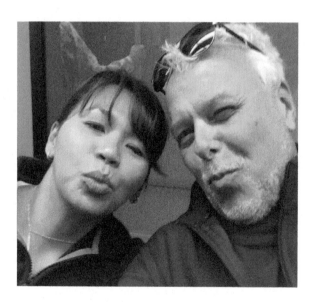

"No end. No beginning.

Only today."

(Ken Ballard, 2023)

Table of Contents

Intro

A somber but important reminder that each of us dissociates from every day.

We are all terminal.

Whether the end comes today, overnight, six months, or many years from now. There will be an end.

How many times do we say when I retire I will (fill in the blank)? Or when I lose 20 lbs. I will (fill in the blank). Wait too long and we lose our chance to fill in the blanks. Stop treating tomorrows like they are limitless. They're not. They are very, VERY finite. We just don't know the exact number ahead of us and in many cases, won't know that number until we've already or are about to run out of them. And some of us may find out how long and then start to plan on a very limited time budget.

PLEASE just start living today. It's easy. Let me help you ask yourself, "and what exactly are you waiting for again?" I am a two-time pancreatic cancer survivor. One day that sentence will be true, but ONLY in the past tense.   In dealing with this disease, I found that the best strategy has been to get to and stay in a place of **absolute humility**. No entitlement. No righteousness. No denial. No arrogance or self-centeredness or anger. Just being and staying humble. And it can be an ongoing journey. Anger and sadness and feeling cheated don't just magically drop away. Humility takes time and work. I'm not here to preach. There is no gospel to be found in these pages. I would like to simply remind us of one simple truth. The end will eventually come. Enjoy your life before it does.

So here are my thoughts on living through and after a health crisis. And even if you are healthy, you may have awoken this morning and found yourself all of a sudden, a more senior person than you had ever realized. There is still time left to look back and say that you are happy with the way you have lived and will keep living. This world is not and has never been about you. But your life and how you live it is entirely and exclusively about you.

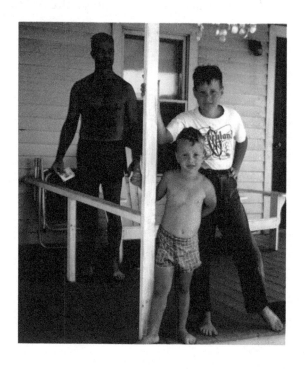

About the book title? Yesterday was New Year's Eve 2022. I had spent another year cancer free, God willing. From the day of my birth through yesterday, I had lived 22,731 days. New Year's Day today would bring me up to 22,732.

The title simply celebrates my "tomorrow". That day we are not ever guaranteed but need to keep in our cross-hairs to help us keep going. Even when it is really, REALLY hard, whatever the struggle we are experiencing that is making it difficult. Staying positive can be the only way forward.

<u>Chapter 1 - Why Me?</u>

Try not to spend too much time trying to figure this out. It's not very helpful. This applies to cancer or any other bad thing that did or can happen to you. Just remember every day, that you didn't ask for it. Say that again. **You did not ask for it.** Bad things happen to good people and are not tied to the consequences of their behavior.

When I was 11 years old someone stole my bicycle. I lamented to a friend "why me"? He asked me what was it that I was really saying? Was I asking why not someone else instead of me and was I wishing my ill fortune on that nameless person? He really pissed me off. I was not wishing my bad luck on ANYONE. Just not on me. I guess some 50 years later my response to him is that I just felt REALLY bad that I was the random victim of a bicycle thief and that I did not need a self-righteous lecture. Just acknowledgement that it sucked and that I felt bad.

So, with my cancer diagnosis I have asked myself:

- Was it genetic?

- Was it environmental pollution?

- Did I not exercise better health habits?

- And the most important question of all regarding the first three questions: What does it really matter?

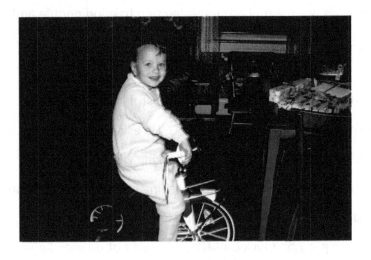

Don't play the "it wasn't my fault" game. Whatever the reason, we still got to this place and again, and I can't repeat this enough, we DIDN'T ask to be here. But we need a path forward. Even if we could assign probabilities to the causes, how does that really help NOW? Right. It doesn't. And for the record, I wish like hell that this didn't happen to me. But I wish even more that it would **NEVER, EVER** happen to anyone. I just never, ever want my life, or my bicycle stolen.

Chapter 2 – Faith

This is the part about death and dying. And how you feel about it. Few of us really want to anticipate what it's like. I don't. I'm scared to death of it. I'm 60. But I ask myself would I be less afraid if I were 90? Answer? No. That is pretty much why I won't live in fear and obsess over it, throughout my remaining days. Time enough to be afraid of death when I'm 90, if I am lucky enough to get there. I don't need a long head start on fear or worrying.

But faith, whatever yours may be, can be immensely helpful and comforting. Do we really know what, if anything, awaits us in an afterlife? If you have your doubts like me, then your answer is no, we don't really know. But if you have faith, then you believe with absolute certainty in whatever you have your faith. That's a great asset. Don't wait to embrace that faith. Let it comfort and guide you. Without it, the process of death and dying becomes much harder.

As for me, I hope for my final moment in this life to be one in which I experience the communal brotherhood of every living thing that has ever lived anywhere. Meaning we ALL have to go sometime. We are all <u>uniquely special</u> but ultimately <u>no different</u> in death and dying from each other.

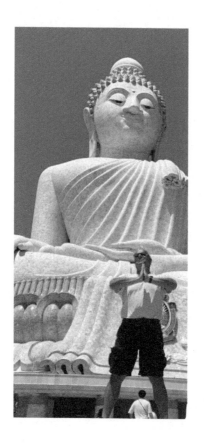

And then I hope for a beyond that renders death truly insignificant and unremarkable in comparison to the absolute grandeur that follows. With all my being, I hope for that.

Chapter 3 – Grace

I have been frequently told throughout my health "journey" by my friends watching my struggle, that I am the most courageous and gracious person they have ever met. Thank you. And by the way, I don't know what that means.

Courage, I think I understand. Most of the time it means either fighting furiously or keeping your lip from trembling when you're dreadfully afraid.

But what exactly is Grace?

Is it accepting eventual defeat without acting like a baby?

Is it believing in divine intervention and giving over control to a divine being?

Does it mean just trying to act cool with it all, when you are really pissed-off?

To me Grace means humility. It means believing that we are all equal. No one grander than the next. It means knowing, again, that I didn't ask for this but that it is the hand I must play. It means not being a jerk and acting-out against others to somehow vent my feelings that this is totally unfair. It means standing against those who want to insulate their own vulnerability against the same fate by believing they, in some way, are special and it could never happen to them. But prior to about eight years ago I neither would have placed my name and the word cancer in the same sentence.

Grace means sucking it up but not without a quiet, relentless fight. Grace also means remaining grateful for all of the days and good fortune behind me and unashamedly asking for more tomorrows ahead of me.

Grace is knowing that I have the right to be here and that I have been and always will be in this life, a guest and cotenant on a term lease. But I've paid my rent and I will stay here as long as I am able. Without apology.

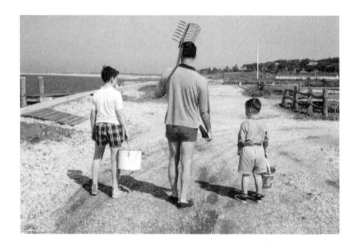

And finally, grace is realizing at long last, that whatever is happening, I have absolutely no control over it whatsoever. And regardless of how I may actually feel about that, I just accept it. And commit to moving forward.

<u>Chapter 4 – Hope</u>

When we are young, we dream and hope big. When we get older, we reach for smaller hopes on a more limited scope.

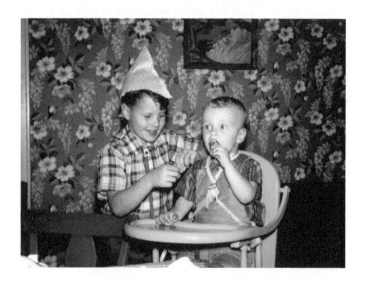

I say this because I have a circle of friends who are also fighting this disease. Sometimes we go from hoping that the cancer will go away, to hoping that it won't get any worse. Or that it won't hurt too much. And sometimes just hoping for a "good" day and trying not to feel defeated when that "feeling better" day does not come exactly when we ask for or need it.

Hope is a great tool for motivation, for positivity, for getting past the really bad moments. Sometimes it's hard to find. Other times I just need to grab onto it and let it lead me forward. But it's what we need as humans. Find hope wherever you can and whenever you need it. And know that you may not always get what you hope for exactly at that moment in time you expect or want it. But don't ever let that defeat your hope.

Chapter 5 - The Truly Unwelcomed and Uninvited

I'm not sure if this will help anyone sort out getting the bad news of a possibly terminal condition, but here goes.

When I got word that my cancer had come back silently, I freaked out. I guess it was the first time I really had to face a shorter life. I had spent my first cancer in denial. That it must have been some kind of freak mistake and that it couldn't possibly ever happen again. Hmmmm. And the second time it was completely unexpected because, unlike the first time, I was in the best health of my life (I felt) and completely on top of my game (I thought).

Cancer really can be an unwelcome and uninvited guest. But more than anything it is completely unexpected. I didn't see it coming and worse, once here, there was no way of knowing where it would take me. And I still don't.

I grew up knowing cerebrally that life is short and its path uncertain and unpredictable. But we seduce ourselves into thinking it is relatively certain and predictable. Until something happens that reminds us that it isn't. I'm not at all happy about this.

Chapter 6 - Tick, Tick, Tick

I'm living in the aftermath of successful cancer treatment. Twice. And then again, I'm waiting...

Is it just the calm between the storms or is the maelstrom really over this time? And since the end comes to us all, is worrying about it even a productive use of my time?

Like "falling off the wagon", when you end your last cancer treatment, the clock resets to zero and you start adding up the days again. The myth is that the further away from zero you get the lower your chances of some kind of relapse. Yea, that may be truly a myth, but as long as I believe it, it helps me keep going.

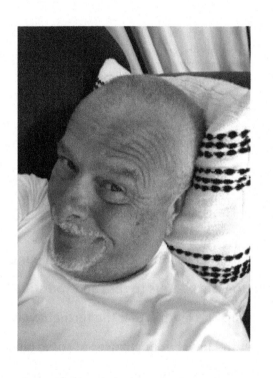

Chapter 7 - Carpe Diem

No matter how we live, one day we will be gone. We will only be making the grass grow greener or our ashes will be forever dispersing across the planet.

Let today be your gift to yourself. It is your one sure thing. Carpe diem.

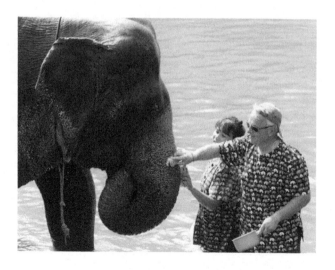

Chapter 8 - Measuring Success

At the end of your life how will you have measured your own success? Will it be how much money you earned? How much you saved and passed along to your survivors? Will it be how high you climbed in your career or organization?

Or will it be something less tangible? Like how many people loved you and called you friend and I'm not talking about the number on your social media page. Will it be how much love and kindness you spread around during your life? Will it be how many friends checked in with you when you were sick? Or most supremely, how you feel about yourself?

If your measurement is about money and wealth, or organizational stature, what happens if those things go away tomorrow, through recession or downsizing or because you are now too expensive for your organization? Or for a myriad of other reasons for unexpected or undeserved change?

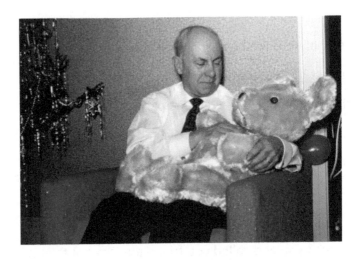

Or will you be able to say that the love and kindness you gave, are the true worth of your character and measure of your life success? If not, there's still time to help make the world a healing place for others.

Chapter 9 - The Time You Have Left is Your Own

This, more than anything else you will read in this book, needs your attention. Your time, however long, or shorter than you had anticipated, is STILL your own. All the way forward. So, you can fill your remaining time with habitual behaviors and actions. Or you can decide to do the things that you don't want to think about in your very last moments, wishing that you had done them, but damn... you didn't.

Yeah, we all have commitments and many of those are rewarding. But maybe go through the exercise of listing out all the things that you insist that you have to do on a regular basis, and then start lining some of them out. And then promise yourself that you will not write them back in later. And promise yourself that when you catch yourself doing them, you will stop.

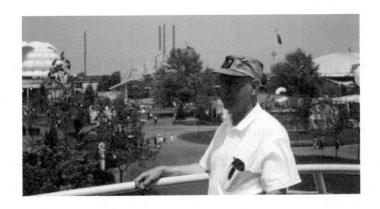

Now go ahead and read that list. Slowly. Does it in any way look like the things you enjoy doing? Or is it a list of habits which you just do because, well, they "need to be done"? Old habits are hard to break. Just try to catch yourself and remember, this may not be how you want to play out your remaining days.

<u>Chapter 10 - Make that List of Everything</u>
<u>You Would Do if You Won the Lottery</u>

Got that list ready and in hand?

OK, I'm sorry to tell you, but you didn't win. But go ahead and do some of those things anyway. Granted that some may involve what you would do with a lot of money. But pick a few things that really are not dependent upon a financial windfall and go ahead and try doing those things. Or try one thing. This is the time for you to NOT use money as an excuse for NOT living.

But if you find that it's not fun, then PLEASE stop. If you like to read, and after the first chapter it just doesn't grab you, for God's sake stop reading. If you like television or movies and you're only watching a show and are quietly saying to yourself, I hope that it will get better? Stop watching. Remember, there are lots of books and television shows and movies to watch and don't be OCD about finishing what you start, especially when you know you're not liking it. The time you have left is truly your own. Don't let old habits run out your clock.

Chapter 11 - Keep Planning for Tomorrow

Plan your tomorrows because it keeps you engaged in your future. And that involvement brings most of us joy. Whether routine chores, or a day trip or a DIY project. Or a longer-range project or travel or anything else goal-oriented. It lets you feel and believe that your tomorrows are still your own. They are. There is nothing sadder or emptier to reflect upon than a today with no tomorrow following it. Stay involved in planning your every tomorrow.

Plan. It feels good.

But there is a trap to avoid. Please don't always "look forward" to avoid showing up and living in the present. My father was notorious for that. Spent each of his annual summer vacation trips talking about the next vacation, totaling evaporating his current vacation fun into a future that wasn't guaranteed. Sadly, he really only succeeded in never being fully in the moment to actually enjoy even one of his present vacations.

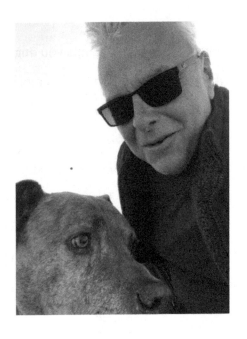

Here's another rule: When you show up to your day, be all there and all in.

Chapter 12 - Endorphins Heal, Cortisol Kills

For your own sake, be happy like your life depends upon it. Because it does.

I'm not saying that living with a terminal or chronic illness is joyful. Never deny how badly you feel. How unfair it feels. How scared you feel. But let yourself feel all of that and let it play out to the fullest, until you are exhausted from feeling bad. You ever find yourself dwelling on something negative and then after a while you say to yourself, "All right, stop! I'm tired of feeling bad?" Or, "I'm exhausted from being in this funk?" Right. Your body is telling you to move past it, by producing its own pain-relieving hormones and neurotransmitters. Let them work for you. If you steep yourself in sadness and stubbornly cling to it, your body will kill you prematurely from the inside out. Be your own best friend and once you are so damn tired of being in a funk, then finally let yourself start to feel good again. Even if this all seems counterintuitive.

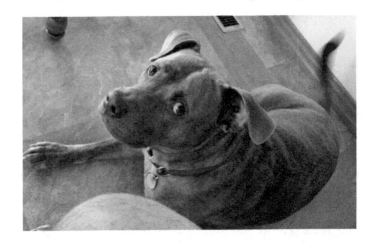

And know that you will repeat this cycle many times. But come out of the darkness however you are able. Sunlight on your face ALWAYS feels good.

Friends going through the same battle tell me that positivity is my best medicine. It's probably because negativity turns out to be the worst toxin. Please believe this.

<u>Chapter 13 - Procrastinating the Bad</u>

Go ahead and do that. Why do today what you can put off until tomorrow? Especially if it's unpleasant and you don't want to do it. And the joy in learning tomorrow that it didn't need to be done and you didn't slog through something unnecessary and waste time? Very cool!

And if it just sits on a nagging to do list, and there's no real harm in removing it, then remove it and stop thinking about it.

Chapter 14 - Procrastinating the Good?
Why Wait to Reward Yourself?

Don't do that. You can inadvertently raise the bar too high and you will never allow yourself the good, fun and nice things in life. Why even have a bar to raise? This is probably residual to your childhood: "You can't have that special thing until you've done something worthy."

Well, you are worthy. Give yourself something special. No strings or conditions attached.

Don't get me wrong. Doing something worthy is a good thing. Just untie it from the reward. The two can be disconnected. Don't put off rewarding yourself.

So, order that lobster or chocolate cake. Get a spa treatment. Get a pedicure or a massage. Take a road trip with an old friend or a new pet. You are good enough and have done enough good deeds in life. Be good to yourself.

Chapter 15 - Take the Plastic Covers Off of the Couch and Use the Good China

If you don't, someone else will when you are gone. Or worse, they will sell them on your front lawn for next to nothing, to clear out your house. Or even worse still, toss them all in the trash and then no one you care about ever got to enjoy them. Waiting for the good company?

YOU are the good company.

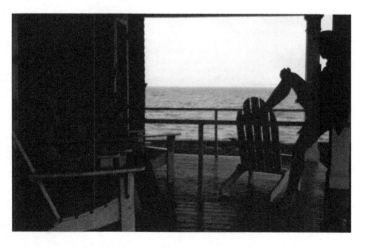

Chapter 16 - Get it Off Your Chest

Is not speaking your mind to someone about keeping your internal peace or more about preserving your relationship with him or her?

If it's about keeping your internal peace, I totally get it. Sometimes getting yourself fired-up is more damaging to yourself. But if you are preserving a relationship which might be damaged by speaking your mind then ask yourself . . . what exactly are you preserving? Maybe you can keep it positive and retool the relationship. But if you can't, don't worry about it, because maybe it wasn't worth preserving.

This is not about giving yourself permission to shoot off your mouth to everybody who walks on your lawn. It's about NOT carrying a burden no one asked you to carry and will eventually wear you out. And after you are gone, no one will really care about anything that ever bothered you. Don't be a martyr and carry the weight of some slight or grievance that happened a long time ago, that no one else remembers.

<u>Chapter 17 - Being Judgmental</u>

Like it or not we are all judgmental. Just try to hold off on being judgmental as long as possible. When you think you have someone's number, remind yourself that you haven't walked in their shoes and can't even begin to know about the battles they are fighting.

Your judgment is only your own private conclusion, right or wrong. You don't get points or a prize for being right. People are who they are and this can be personally disappointing, but only if you let it. Don't let it.

Chapter 18 - Forgive or Forget

One is emotional, one is cognitive. And it may be impossible to do both. Again, remember that carrying that old grievance only hurts you. Most people really don't care or consider how you feel about them. You are not punishing them with your silent anger. You're really only hurting yourself. Let it go. Don't get an ulcer or cancer by eating yourself alive. I'll try to say this as nicely as possible:

Only very few people really care. For the rest, it's not personal.

Spend your energy caring about yourself, your happiness, your health and all of those things for those you love. Please don't carry the weight of the memories or grievances that the world has not stopped to give a second thought.

And don't overthink this, or for that matter, anything else. By doing so we throw away the genetic gifts from our ancestors of instincts and gut feelings. Those gifts we received through our DNA so we wouldn't need to relearn literally EVERYTHING with every new generation. Sadly, our cerebral cortex just makes us dwell on stuff in an endless loop, and most of the time we find ourselves back to where out instincts would have led us.

So, think about that, but try not to overthink it. LOL

Chapter 19 - Receiving Advice

Some people just listen and are completely supportive to your opinion? Most people, <u>right</u>? Yea... no.

Lots of people, for their own sake and not yours, need to be heard, validated, be provocative, or show everyone how smart they are. What better person than to someone (you) who has just given them an opening to "opinionate"?

I've learned from experience who to pull into my own decision-making process. Those people are very few and don't jump right in without invitation. The people I choose to help me sort things out are <u>some </u>family members, not all, and <u>certain</u> friends, again, not all. And those people know me well and know I don't appreciate anything unsolicited.

The truly helpful person doesn't start out by telling you what they would do in your place. They generally ask questions to help you decide what you want to do in your place and withhold their opinion. Just be careful about who you invite to help and don't be afraid to tell someone to save their breath. You can do it nicely.

Chapter 20 – Being Kind isn't a Chore or Favor

Don't argue with this one. Do a good deed. If you pick someone who isn't grateful, don't give them your time or kindness again. Very few people are jerks, but there are jerks out there. Just <u>don't stop</u> being kind to others. Just to the jerks.

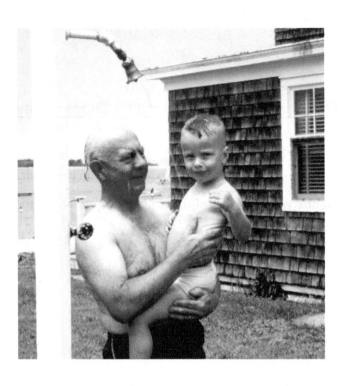

Wouldn't it be nice if the whole world paid their gratitude forward? Instead of exacting their revenge for old faceless anger forward?

Chapter 21 – Saying No

It's not rude to say no. Just politely explain that you can't help someone with THAT whatever THAT happens to be. Tell them it's not a good time. And you will let them know when it is a good time. Most of us don't like being put on the spot.

No more details. The more you don't feel like saying yes, and the more you make excuses about it, the more ridiculous you appear. Remember it's your time that you are guarding and you have the right to do so.

Chapter 22 - Bad Relationships

This is a big one. Are you are already envisioning the end of a relationship? Do you instinctively know that you're done with somebody and are looking for a door? Then suck it up now and end it. Who in this life is the only person that you can rely upon to ensure your happiness? Yea. You. And if you mess this one up and permit one more year or month or day with someone who you can't imagine being with until the end? Well, you have failed the most basic responsibility you have over your own life: to make yourself happy.

Chapter 23 - Stop Reliving the Past

You can't change yesterday. Why dwell on what you should have done, unless it is a path forward not to make the same mistake again? Just trust you won't. Don't rehearse in your creative memory how you would have stood up for yourself 50 years ago, but didn't. Just do it next time.

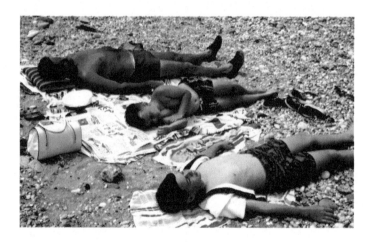

<u>Chapter 24 - Finishing that To Do List</u>

The day after my Aunt Eveline passed away in 1998, I noticed something that has always stayed with me. She was a huge fan of doing needlepoints. On a frame next to her bed was one that was only half-completed. I took it off of the frame and to this day it hangs in my bathroom to remind me that there will always be something we leave undone.

Come to think of it there was a paperback book next to her bed with a bookmark halfway through the pages. There was laundry in a pile she had intended to wash. There were dirty dishes in her sink. There was a myriad of day-to-day tasks and projects which permanently became frozen in time.

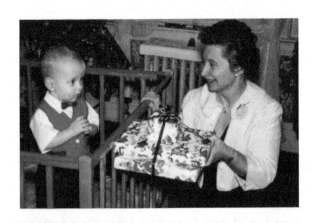

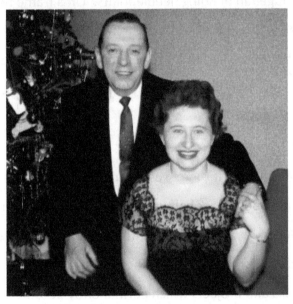

I'm fairly OCD. I love my lists and checking off what I've done. I have to admit leaving stuff undone behind me is unsettling. I just need to be settled with the knowledge that there will always be stuff I never get to complete.

But I need to just let those things be routine and unimportant. But also, to make sure the important stuff is done and settled. Beneficiary designations. Wills. Access to online accounts. Passwords. Trusts. Putting down on paper what I want. Witnessed. Notarized. If you love your survivors, do them a favor and make sure you make those wishes memorialized and legal. It will cause them huge headaches if you don't.

Quick story. I knew a woman who passed away a few years ago and she was obsessed with changing her last will and testament every few months, every time someone crossed her and she wanted to exact a "post-mortem" retaliation. I thought it was petty but that was entirely her business.

The irony to the story is that she was in the middle of making major changes to her will, yet again, and then died suddenly. What stopped her from finalizing that last will was a dispute with her attorney over the attorney fees involved in making minor changes. The amount was truly nominal, but that disagreement resulted in a whole bunch of people benefitting or not, in a way that in the end she had not intended.

Sad.

Chapter 25 - Write it Down

If it's in your head and you want it out there, write it
down. Post it. Blog it. Publish it. Email it. Text it.

I'm writing this collection of thoughts because if I don't,
one day they will die with me. I'm hoping that some
karma may be shared across the divide between now and
then, by simply getting my thoughts on paper. My hope is
that they may be helpful to someone now.

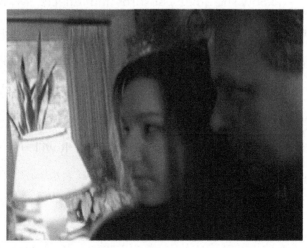

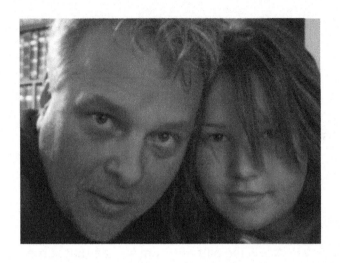

I have no kids, but my niece Katie has enough "Uncle Ken-isms" to get her through some of life's major hurdles. And my niece Kelly, cares even less for unsolicited advice than do I, but I know she quietly absorbs and reflects. My hope is that they both take away from me, by my own behavior or example, something useful. I love you both to death and beyond. People learn mostly by listening or watching, not by talking. But you have your own wisdom. Your cynicism. Your kindness. Get it out there. It will absolutely be helpful to someone.

<u>Chapter 26 - Getting Therapy</u>

Think you are too old? Afraid of the pain that lives just below the surface or content to just go on pretending it's not there? Been successful (somewhat) in keeping it partially buried? Don't have the time because you got this far anyway without professional help?

Therapy is tough. It makes you face your own past, which is often painful and seldom pretty.   Just know that your goal is to be nice to that little child inside of you who got hobbled as a kid.   And know that it wasn't your fault. But it is your responsibility to fix now. However old you are. And what worthier goal is there?

You never, really grow out of a dysfunctional and/or abusive upbringing. That experience becomes your permanent mirror throughout life. But at some point, you learn not to look into that mirror, as the reflection never changes. And you start to look for a new window from which to view the world and your rightful, legitimate place in it.

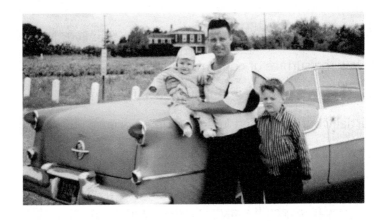

Those scars remain. Therapy will never completely remove them or cure you. But know that you will come out on the other side, a stronger, more confident person and you will stop blaming yourself. And that little kid inside of you will finally realize that it is never too late to have a happy childhood.

Chapter 27 - Adopt that Shelter Pet

Think that caring for a four-legged furry animal is too tough? Or that lowering your blood pressure and increasing your daily dose of joy isn't worth it? Really?

Caring for an animal, as well as you would care for your own child, is hard work. If you're not up to it, then don't do it. You probably already know whether you are a "pet" person. It's a simple test. Does seeing dogs or cats on social media make you go "awwwwww" and make your heart feel all warm and fuzzy? Then step right up. But if those same pictures make you roll your eyes, then don't go there.

Talk to shelter staff. I am a shelter volunteer and our goal is NOT to push pets out to the wrong homes. We will help you go over all of the reasons why you perhaps should NOT adopt. As well as helping you consider the positives. And then just realize that animals, like human beings, take time to adjust to change, especially as they age. Make the commitment if you can. But realize that the rewards, especially the love from that animal, may also take some time to realize. Their love will come when they trust your love and feel less afraid.

And nothing feels better than when that scared, reclusive animal eventually sneaks up next to you and gives you that quick, wet dog lick or cat nuzzle. It doesn't ever get much better than that.

A shout out to the Volunteers of the Burbank Animal Shelter. Their decision to include me on their volunteer staff, putting their trust in me as handler/custodian of their residents, has gotten me through some really tough moments.

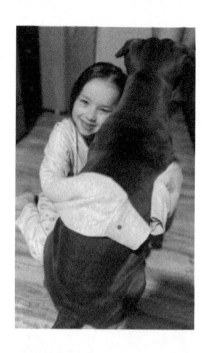

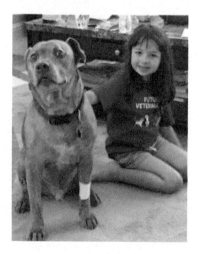

Chapter 28 – Put Down You're Phone

Especially if it's draining your time. How much value is it really adding to your life? Do those little alerts really notify you of something important? Are those suggested videos, contacts, etc., even relevant? Some algorithm somewhere, which you had no input in creating, seems to think so.

You decide. Not your phone or a marketing algorithm. Just do what works for you. Either give yourself a phone-free time every day, and I don't mean while you're asleep at night. Or go cold turkey for a while. You may have to go slow and not expect too much of yourself at first. Addictions are hard to break.

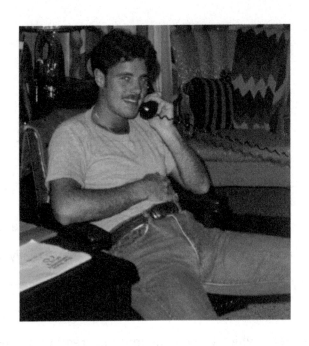

I'm not trying to take away something fun. Just know that if you really look at your time as limited, is this how you really want to spend it? Would you rather be spending it with family, friends and pets? Reading a book? Working out? Road tripping? Hiking? DIY stuff?

Your phone may be stealing that time.

<u>Chapter 29 – God Willing</u>

I end a lot of sentences lately with the words, "God willing".

Does this mean I believe in God? Maybe I do. Or maybe I did. Or maybe I will.

But when I say God willing, what I mean is that I'm not entitled, and I hope for a stroke of faith or luck or divine intervention that will carry me through another day.

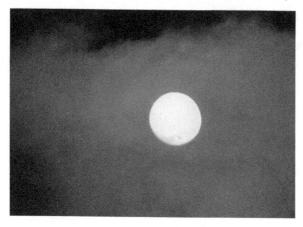

Sometimes I find myself thinking that maybe we were not created by God, in as much as we are quite simply his expression. That all matter and energy, dark and light, are just his constant, unrelenting, unfolding expression of his own existence. Simply, that God didn't create everything, in as much as GOD IS EVERYTHING.

This perspective really does justify being kind to each other considering that through malevolence we destroy a part of Him. I draw great comfort in thinking that I'm not flying solo looking for Him, praying to Him, but that I am actually just a very tiny, yet significant part of Him. Makes me want to be a better person out of sheer gratitude to the part of Him that I represent. Namaste.

Chapter 30 – Entitlement

It really doesn't exist. You may think it does, but it doesn't. Our legal system apparently provides a vehicle for pretty much anybody to challenge your safe haven of entitlement.   Or worse, the older some get, the more they become bigger jerks and full of themselves and convinced that they can do things simply because they can and there are no guard rails.

So, when you hear yourself saying, well "this was a social contract". Or "I worked for this and everybody understood that this is what I get"? Remember, you are only entitled as long as others believe it too. And they may not believe it.

Chapter 31 – Reconnect with Old Friends

Their time is getting shorter also. I get more love and support from the friends I've had since somewhere between age 6 and 20 than many friends from more recent years. I'm finding those friends from long ago wake up memories I'd long forgotten and make me laugh. Or cry. They remind me that they were there and shared many of the moments I had long stored away.

In no particular order, thank you Joe & Lynn, Shari B, Marla F, Sobby & Susie, Sondra W, Andrea T, Howie W, Dave & Kathy F, Kathy H, Larry K, Heidhy M, Phyllis E, Lisa/Alyssa M, Lorrie F, Donna F, Deirdre M, Henry O, Yul E, Michael B, (Mrs.) Sheila Stern (RIP), Debbie F, Marie S, Cindy (RIP) & Joe E, Millie B, Dave (RIP) & Beverly, Patty M, Michele & Mishelle, Phil S, Anna M, Craig M (RIP), MaBel A, Yolanda S, Santa R, Sherrie T, Todd R, Marilou M, Yvette E, Josh S, Christa M, Jesse S, Telly B, Vinnie D, Joey L, Dale L (RIP),

Alison S, Rev Eddie A, Ann D, Noreen S, Gerry A, Mel S, Marion K, Shel K, Tim C, Sylvia G, Elissa G, Mike G (RIP), Katie B, Kelly B, Peggy H, Gloria (GG), Renata O, Jey J, Deb P, Elisabeth O, Lorry I, Pat B, Rodney L, Sue KS, Mrs. Sheila C, Patty R, Pam C, Terry VG, Joanie R, Bev & Ken D, Lynda O, Clarisse C, Omar R, Eleanor O, Bruce B (RIP), Patti WH, Deb C, Robin C, Issy S, Rosa O, Julie B, Aaron W, Ed C, Sue & Jane, Ro C, Molly L, Liz W, Steve G, Ivette Q, Vicki R, Frankie L, Leslie R, Roanne & Edbel, Sunny E, Jeff & Lynn, Izzy C, Rose & Evie C, Jan B, Vinnie S, Ang C, Phyllis C, Steph-Nat-& Mrs. S, Mary & Roger B, Sue S, Dan K, Larry M, Cheryl K, Mary B, Marion F, Gene P, Ben C, Richie G, Judy RL, Terry DG, Sam H, Linda R, Janet G, Steve F, Heather & Buggie M, and my super cool sister in law and newly inducted sister in this survivor's club, Rina E (You Rock!)...

The list goes on. If I never said it exactly like this, to all of you, "thank you all for your friendship." It's the one thing in life I truly got to hang on to and take along with me for this unbelievably magnificent ride.

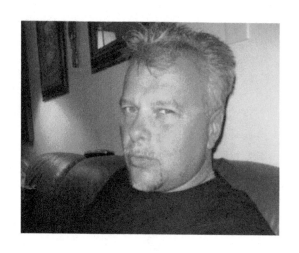

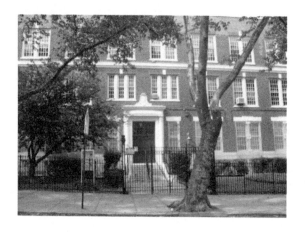

Chapter 32 – Poetic Injustice

Some random thoughts from a guy (me) who refuses to be run over:

*   *   *   *   *

It's the dark shoe that falls when you're not looking

You don't hear it

After it's fallen you may not even notice

Cancer reminds you daily that the end comes to us all

For some sooner perhaps than later

*   *   *   *   *

Friends ask me how I deal with the prospect of a shorter life

I don't know how to answer except

In the same way they do

only more urgently

*   *   *   *   *

The minute I think I won't beat cancer, the fight is over

I literally must believe that I will prevail until the end many

years from now

Otherwise, there is no point in continuing

*   *   *   *   *

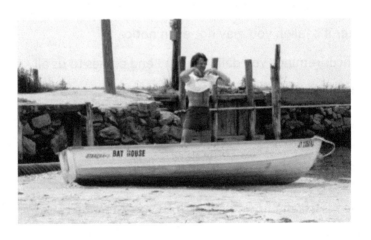

*　　　*　　　*　　　*　　　*

I'm told to fight the good fight

I ask is there really any other kind of fight

*　　　*　　　*　　　*　　　*

I won't let cancer define who I am or was

I would like to be remembered for my friendship, humor

and kindness

And for stomping the crap out of cancer as many times as

necessary

<u>Chapter 33 – The Turtle, the Seagull and the Snail</u>

These were three innocent lives I remember snuffing out quite by accident. Two with my car, one with (don't ask) a garbage disposal. I guarantee that none of them knew me or could in any way identify the arbiter of their fates. But I remember each event vividly with sadness and remorse, across many years between then and now. No other human will ever know or remember these creatures, whose lives I myself extinguished through mindless carelessness. I never got to tell them that I was sorry. They wouldn't have understood me if I had.

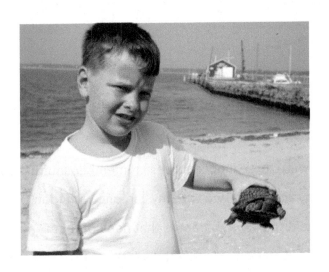

But I say today, I'm so very sorry to each of you.

So please. Don't kill thoughtlessly or needlessly. **It's really so unnecessary**.

<u>Chapter 34 – To Cindy</u>

Just as I finished up writing this book today, I received the sad news that a long-term, very dear friend of mine lost her own battle with cancer this morning. She had entered home hospice a few weeks ago, but even with the anticipation of this moment well in advance, losing a close friend is absolutely the very worst, most helpless feeling I have ever experienced.

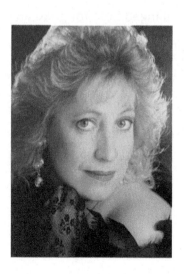

We all lose our cherished connections and as we grow older those losses seem to happen with more frequency, but with no less pain. Those friendships usually sneak up on us silently, almost unnoticed, but when they leave, the hollow echo of that empty space they once occupied is deafening.

Cindy, I close my eyes and hear your infectious laugh. I remember your words which remind me of your razor-sharp humor. In many conversations throughout the years, I remember feeling your kindest of hearts through the phone or across your kitchen table. Your life touched mine and left it changed both for good and for the good. Rest in peace Cin. I will miss you every day going forward without you. If I too lose this fight, please arrange to meet and greet me in my own passing. I trust no friend more than you to show me around.

Chapter 35 – To Doug

I miss my older brother Doug, my one and only biological sibling. He was funny. He was sometimes selfish and self-centered. He was kind. He was full of hope. He was hopeless. He lived life large. He died in a flicker few people noticed. Eighteen years now and I still hear the news from his wife in my head. Like being stabbed with a knife, and feeling the pain of the entry wound, but never really being able to ever pull it out again.

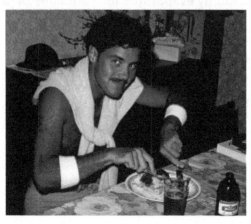

When his wife Gloria was about to lose her own fight with cancer, the technician who delivered the hospice bed to the house asked me if she was related to Doug Ballard. I told him that he was her deceased husband and my brother. The tech had read in a 2004 Sacramento newspaper that Doug had died and always wondered about the back story. He had worked with Doug briefly and always remembered how Doug would always brag to him about his two young daughters. In that moment, I had Doug's oldest daughter Katie, come downstairs to say hello. Funny how the space in between a father's proud stories of his 7-year-old daughter and the adult 24-year-old Katie instantly evaporated into the same person. Somehow, I still feel that Doug was in some way responsible for that moment and meeting.

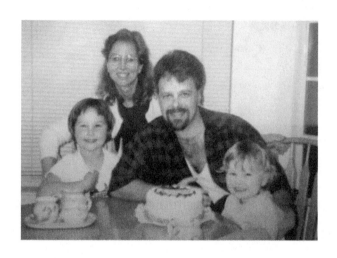

Hey Doug, you had a wonderful wife and two beautiful daughters. But I understand our dysfunctional family growing up and our early years together. I was there and I lived it as well, right alongside of you. That family and those years were mine as well as yours. For good or bad, they made us who we became.

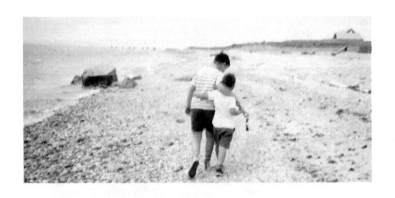

See you on the other side brother. I hope many, **MANY** years from now. I love you then, now and always.

Chapter 36 – To My Friends from Long Ago

I remain grateful and blessed for those of you who take the time out on Facebook to wish me a happy birthday. Or those who go onto the dinosaur of email and write to me about their lives. Or reminisce about old silly memories with me.

I'm sitting here a day before the end of the year. A year that saw me in the bulk of my most recent chemo, and also unsure of whether or not I was going to pull through this time. Well, I pulled through again and remain humble as to how long it will be, if and when I face this again. I sit here with my old dog next to me grateful that I may be able, God willing, I said it again, to live long enough to put him to rest, and not the reverse. Grateful that I feel good and not sick every day. Grateful that I got off of a video call last night with my grade school friends from over 50 years ago. Grateful that I'm waiting for my wife to come home from work, always with hugs and kisses.

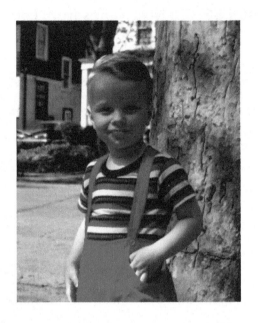

I know that for all of us this world does not last forever. And one day it does end. But I'm happy for now that apparently, I'll be here a little bit longer.

Chapter 37 – To My Wife and Dog

What they do for me is simple. It is **not** necessarily a specific act of kindness or necessarily how they do or don't feel about me. My gratitude comes from my own experience of pure joy and peace and above all, **belonging**, when I am with them. That at this moment in time and space, I am exactly where I am supposed to be. For that I am grateful beyond any words I can think of writing.

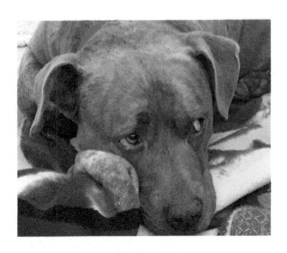

Chapter 38 – Letting the World Go On Without You

This passage more than any other, is the hardest to write. It really comes down to thinking about the time after I'm gone. The world without me. How beautiful the sunrise may be the day after I leave and I'll never see it. It forces me to accept that there will be a time when my influence is over. Put that time far enough ahead in the future and I don't have to think too much about it. But the sooner that reality looms in my mind, the more real and stark it becomes.

I look at my aging dog and pray that he goes before me. Not that my wife won't be absolutely wonderful at taking care of him. She will. I just don't want to think about him wandering around the house, following my ever-dwindling scent and never finding me.

I look at my wife and feel cheated that I may never live to see how beautiful she will be in her old age. I grieve all of the fun we may have had but no longer will. I worry about not being here to protect her, to make her laugh, to feel my loving touch. I worry about her sorrow and how it will affect her health. I don't worry that she may go on and find ways to be happy. This is what I hope most for her. With all my heart. It is just painfully sad that I would no longer be a part of it.

How do I deal with it? Not very well. It's waves of sadness and anger and fear. It's knowing that whatever I do now in advance of an end, won't provide for every last thing my wife and dog will ever need.

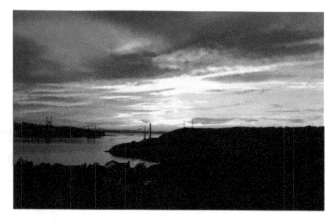

I therefore choose to do <u>now</u> whatever I want to do <u>now</u> to enjoy my remaining time. We constantly hear that life is short. However long or short, we have to live it on our own terms and enjoy it as fully as we can. And not worry that we won't get to everything. We won't.

<u>Chapter 39 – Saying Goodbye</u>

This one is easy. I don't say goodbye. But every day I tell those closest to me that I love them and I say it with all my heart. And I make sure that they feel it.

This photo is of my grandparents, Jessie and Paul. It was taken in the late 1950's and I have lived without them since the mid 1990's. I didn't ever get the chance to say goodbye to them really. Silly, since after almost thirty years, not for a single day have they ever really left me.

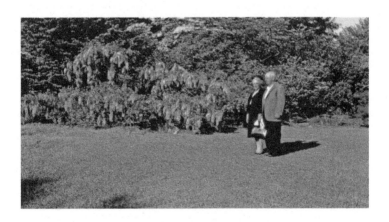

<u>Chapter 40 – Ask Yourself One Last Time</u>

So now that you have spent the last few hours wading through my ramblings, philosophizing and reminiscing, I ask you to do one more thing. Take a minute and answer yourself one question. Whether you're looking down the throat of a possibly terminal illness, or just old age like many of us, what are you going to do with the rest of your day, your week, your year? What exactly is it that you are waiting for?

If your genuine answer is "nothing different", that you've achieved and experienced everything that you wanted to and you're done, then OK. I don't quite believe you, but it's ok to feel like you've done enough. But if you still have more on your plate, more life to pursue, more dreams that you left undone somewhere behind you, then start. Now.

It's never too late. Until it's too late. As I said, you may have to go slow and not expect too much of yourself at first. On ALL of the thoughts I raised in this book. I'm just trying to help you focus on the rest of your life and ways to command control of it. The rest is up to you.

<u>Outro</u>

Here I am spending my limited remaining life doing one of the things that I love most. Hiking at the beach with my best friend Henry, both of us looking ahead toward new tomorrows. Find your own JOY and ENJOY your best life.

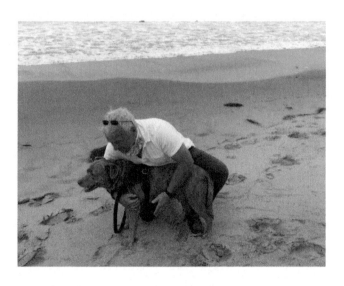

"No end. No beginning. Only today."

(Ken Ballard, 2023)

About the Artist (Gloria Celine Gonzales-Ballard)

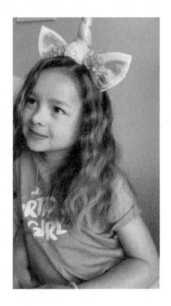

Gloria currently resides in Roseville CA with her mom (Kelly), auntie (Katie) and best doggie friend (Asher Mae). When not pursuing her artistic talents, she is studying to graduate 1st grade, dreaming of a career as a veterinarian and hanging out with her dad, and pals Dej and Peggy.

When asked if she could help out with illustrating the cover of Uncle Ken's book, she laughed, shrugged and assured, "Yea, I'm good with that!" A very special thank you to my favorite young lady, for helping me to remember to bring my very best to every moment, to enjoy today completely and always cherish the next, or in my case, day 22,733. Great job Glo! I love you so very much!

About the Author (Ken Ballard)

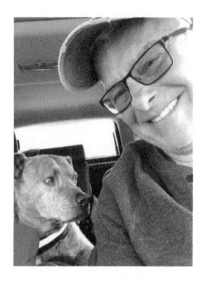

As of this writing Ken is still alive and well, living with his wife Rissa and his wonderful dog (and best friend) Henry. He is retired from Federal Service and volunteers at the Burbank Animal Shelter, many of their temporary residents becoming inspirations for the canine characters in his upcoming book "A Council of Dogs (An Anthology)", scheduled for release in early 2024.

Ken has spent his earlier years playing trumpet and flugelhorn for the Queensborough Symphonic Band, holds his MBA from Baruch College CUNY, has kayaked the Andaman Sea and has driven sled dog teams in Seward, Alaska. As he likes to say, he's "just getting warmed up".

Ken still battles cancer every day, but doesn't wish to make that the one thing he is remembered for. He prefers to be the author who writes in fragments, ends sentences with prepositions, and speaks from his core about animal protection, kindness and love. He hopes that you find something you connect to in any of his passages to be kind enough to share this book on your own social media. He would like his life and writings to provide some level of comfort to those of you who, like him, never thought they would hear their own name and the word cancer in the same sentence. "There may be no way to be completely at peace with it or make sense of it, but you bring your best fight to the battle."

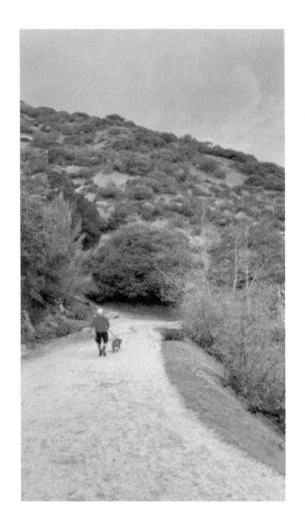

(Los Angeles CA, January 1, 2023)

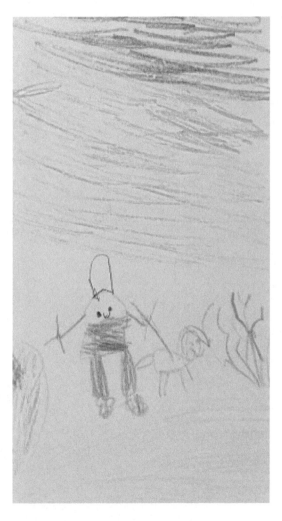

(By Gloria Celine Gonzales-Ballard, July 27, 2023)

Made in the USA
Las Vegas, NV
15 December 2023

82886687R00069